PAMELA D MOORE

When Tomorrow Fades:

The Caregivers Guide to Survival, while Caring for a Loved One with Dementia

Copyright © 2024 by Pamela D Moore

All rights reserved. No part of this publication may be reproduced, stored or transmitted in any form or by any means, electronic, mechanical, photocopying, recording, scanning, or otherwise without written permission from the publisher. It is illegal to copy this book, post it to a website, or distribute it by any other means without permission.

First edition

This book was professionally typeset on Reedsy. Find out more at reedsy.com

Contents

1. Introduction — 1
2. When Life Turns Upside Down and you're told your loved one... — 5
   What is Dementia? How does it compare to normal aging? — 6
   The Different Types of Dementia — 7
3. How Dementia Changes Your Loved One and Yourself -... — 13
   Imagine a Day in the Life of someone with Dementia — 13
   How your loved one behaves' is your Window into the Disease — 15
   Recognizing Needs Beyond Symptoms — 15
   Your Reactions: Finding Grace in the Challenges — 17
   First Steps now you have a Diagnosis — 17
4. Navigating the Maze of What Comes Next? — 24
   Changing How You Communicate — 25
   How to Have a Great Conversation with Your Loved One — 26
   Responding Calmly to Agitation or Repetitive Behaviors — 27
   Understanding Triggers and Behaviors — 27
5. Recognizing the Signs of Late-Stage Dementia — 34
   Physical and Cognitive Changes — 34

Health Complications to Expect	35
Emotional and Spiritual Preparation	36
Engaging Hospice and Palliative Care Services	38
6 Honoring Caregivers'	41
Why Self-Care Matters	42
Recognizing Stress (And What It Does to You)	42
Practical Self-Care Strategies	43
Balancing Care giving and Your Personal Life	44
When You Feel Overwhelmed	45
You Deserve Care, Too	46
7 The Final Goodbye	48
Recognizing End-of-Life Symptoms	48
Honoring Their Legacy	49
Grieving and Healing	51
Rediscovering Your Own Identity	53
Maintaining Your Connection with Them	53
Helping Others on the Journey	54
8 Conclusion: A Journey of Love, Laughter, and Purpose	55
Finding Your Purpose in This New Reality	56
Carrying Their Light Forward	57
Final Thoughts	57
9 Resources	59

1

Introduction

There is a certain irony in how Dementia works. The illness that steals so much from the one we love somehow grants us a peculiar richness if we dare to accept it. It is a thief and a teacher, a heartbreak and a profound blessing all rolled into one. Few journeys demand more of us or offer as many unpolished gems as the road we travel with a loved one, who is, slowly losing their memories—and, in some ways, gaining something else entirely. We begin life needing the care of others and the irony is we end life the same way.

For more than twenty years, I have walked this road as a hospice nurse, alongside families who carried the weight of a Dementia diagnosis. I have sat at kitchen tables where cups of tea grew cold while stories of frustration, exhaustion, anger, and love spilled like rivers. I've helped children become caregivers, spouses learn to redefine love, and friends find their way through the fog of literal and metaphorical confusion. Every family was different, and every story was unique, but the common thread was always this: no one felt prepared for the journey.

How could they? How could you? After all, there's no map for this.

- No tidy set of instructions for how to care for someone who might look the same but is slowly transforming into someone unfamiliar.
- No guidebook for what to do when your father doesn't recognize your face or when your spouse asks to go home while sitting in the living room of the house you built together. There is, however, one thing I can promise you. You don't have to travel this road alone, and though the road may twist and turn, there is beauty to be found along the way!

Let me say this at the outset: **Dementia affects you, too**. It doesn't discriminate between society, rich, poor, or educated. It will test your patience, resolve, humor, and ability to grieve a thousand small losses while still showing up daily with love. It is, in short, one of the hardest things you will ever do. But it is also an invitation—albeit one wrapped in sadness and uncertainty—to discover the depths of your compassion and the unyielding resilience of the human spirit.

I've seen it. Families find joy in the simplest moments—a spontaneous laugh, a touch of the hand, a fleeting but radiant moment of clarity. I've seen caregivers develop a sense of humor so sharp and tender it could pierce through even the thickest clouds of despair when a spouse puts the washing into the fridge, and the food into the washing machine. I've seen grown children learn how to dance to the rhythm of their mother's forgotten songs and spouses who, though bewildered and tired, fall in love all over again with the essence of a person who's still there, even as they change. I've seen close to miracles when someone so shut off and closed down begins to sing when music is played. The video linked below will make even the most hardened of us cry at what can be awakened with touch and a kind voice.

Gladys Wilson and Naomi Feil [Video]. YouTube. https://www.youtube.com/watch?v=CrZXz1oFcVM

And I've seen the other side, too. Days when you feel like you're failing. When guilt and anger wrap around your ankles like chains, and you wonder if you're strong enough for this.

Here's what I want you to know: You are. You don't have to be perfect—no one is. You simply have to show up, as you are, with love, curiosity, and a willingness to learn. The journey will change you, but it does not have to break you.

This book is not a manual. It won't tell you exactly what to do or how to feel—because that would be as impossible as writing a recipe for perfection. What it will do, I hope, is offer you a companion. Someone to walk alongside you as you navigate the waves, someone who understands the peculiar heartbreak of loving someone who is slowly forgetting. Someone to remind you that there is still light, even on the darkest days, and that the moments of connection—no matter how fleeting—are worth treasuring.

When tomorrow fades, as it inevitably will, what remains is the love you bring to this moment, to this day. And as much as Dementia takes, it also leaves behind an extraordinary opportunity: to love more deeply, to laugh more freely, and to live with a raw, unfiltered appreciation for the present.

So, let's begin. Together, we'll explore what it means to care for someone with Dementia—the challenges, the heartbreaks, and the unexpected joys. Let's talk about navigating this uncharted territory, not as a battle to be won, but as a journey to be lived. And perhaps, as we walk this path together, you'll find that, even in the shadow of forgetting, something is amazing, waiting to be discovered.

2

When Life Turns Upside Down and you're told your loved one is diagnosed with Dementia.

Where do you start to Understand the Dementia puzzle?

There is no preparation for the moment when a physician looks at you, tilts their head just slightly, and says words you never thought you'd hear: your loved one has Dementia. It feels as though the world has tilted off its axis. The ground beneath you shifts, and you find yourself in a strange new landscape, where the rules you thought you knew no longer apply.

It's not just a diagnosis; it's a doorway into uncertainty, a million questions tumbling out at once. What does this mean? How will it change them?

How will it change me? And, perhaps most poignantly, how

much time do we have left before the person I love begins to fade?

What is Dementia? How does it compare to normal aging?

To begin navigating this journey, it helps to understand what Dementia is and what it does to the brain.

Dementia is not a single disease; it's an umbrella term that covers several conditions that affect memory, thinking, and behavior. It happens when neurons—the brain's vital communication cells—become damaged and stop functioning properly. Depending on the type of Dementia, this damage can occur in different regions of the brain, leading to distinct symptoms and challenges.

Here's a simplified way to think of it: your brain is like a well-orchestrated piece of music, with each section playing its part to create harmony.

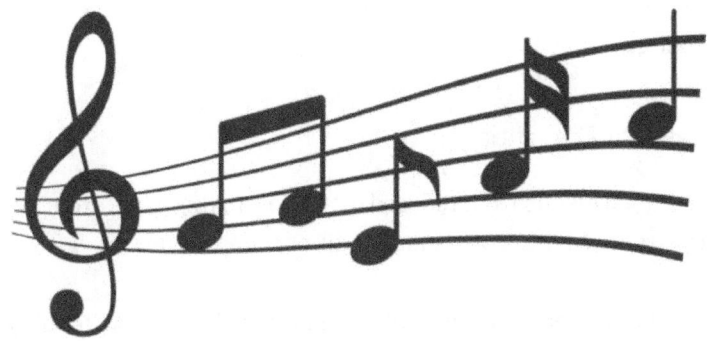

Dementia disrupts this symphony. One section forgets its notes, another plays out of tune, and eventually, the music falters. Over time, this disruption affects more than just memory; it impacts language, reasoning, emotions, and even the ability to perform basic daily tasks.

The Different Types of Dementia

When your loved one receives their diagnosis, the doctor might use terms that feel unfamiliar or overwhelming or just plain foreign. While all forms of Dementia share similarities, there are distinct types:

Alzheimer's Disease

The most common type of Dementia accounts for about 60-80% of cases. It's caused by sticky clumps of tissue and twisted fibers in the brain that block the brain's cells from talking to each other properly.

Memory loss is often the first noticeable symptom, followed

by confusion, difficulty organizing thoughts, and personality changes.

Vascular Dementia

This type results from reduced blood flow to the brain, often due to strokes or other vascular conditions.

Symptoms can vary but might include problems with planning, focus, or walking. It's sometimes described as more "spotty" in its effects, with certain abilities remaining intact while others decline.

Lewy Body Dementia

This type happens when unusual protein clumps called Lewy bodies build up in the brain and disrupt brain function.

It's known for causing visual hallucinations, fluctuating levels of alertness, and movement difficulties (walking, twitching), similar to Parkinson's disease. It's often unpredictable, with good days and bad days.

Frontotemporal Dementia (FTD)

This type affects the frontal and temporal lobes of the brain, which control behavior, language, and decision-making.

Early symptoms often involve personality changes, impulsivity, or difficulty with speech, rather than memory loss.

Normal Pressure Hydrocephalus (NPH)

NPH is a condition where there is a build-up of cerebrospinal fluid (CSF) in the brain's ventricles (fluid-filled spaces). This causes them to enlarge and put pressure on the brain, even though the fluid pressure often appears "normal" during testing.

NPH is often remembered by the "3 W's":

1. **Walking problems** – Trouble walking, with a slow, shuffling, or unsteady gait, like feet are "stuck to the ground."
2. **Memory problems** – Thinking and memory difficulties, which can resemble Dementia.
3. **Urinary issues** – Loss of bladder control or frequent urge to urinate.

These symptoms usually appear gradually and can worsen over time if untreated. In some patients, the symptoms can be reversed after placement of a shunt. My husband was diagnosed with this when he became unable to walk, incontinent, and had sudden and severe difficulty sitting up, eating, and slurring his speech. It took months of doctor visits for them to take him seriously as the symptoms would come and go -always being in remission when we had a doctor's appointment. One day "thankfully" his symptoms appeared as they had him walk to the examination room and they finally saw what we had been seeing as we knew they didn't believe us. The moral here is to keep pushing and not take no for an answer.

Each type of Dementia presents its challenges, and the progression can vary widely from person to person. Understanding the specific diagnosis your loved one has received can help you prepare for what lies ahead and work with their care team to provide the best possible support.

Can You Avoid Catching Dementia?

One of the first fears that often surfaces after a loved one's diagnosis is, *"Will this happen to me?"*

My mother was recently placed in a nursing home having fallen, and for several weeks was terrified and wouldn't leave her room. We struggled to find the cause as this was very unlike her. She finally told my sister she was terrified she would catch Dementia and end up like her neighbor. As my mother has never known anyone with Dementia this was a natural concern. It can be scary if there's a family history of Dementia. Let me put your mind at ease: <u>Dementia is not contagious</u>. You cannot "catch" it from someone; even with close and prolonged care giving.

That said, certain types of Dementia may be genetic, meaning that if a close family member has it, your risk might be slightly higher. However, genetics are just one piece of the puzzle. Lifestyle factors, such as maintaining a healthy diet, staying mentally and physically active, managing stress, and avoiding smoking, are significant in reducing your overall risk.

Think of your brain as a garden. Genetics may determine the kind of soil you've been given, but how you care for that garden—

what you plant, how you water it, and protect it from weeds—makes a tremendous difference. While there are no guarantees, a healthy lifestyle can help support brain health and reduce your risk of cognitive decline.

So what's next?

Receiving a Dementia diagnosis is a seismic event, but it is not the end of the story. It is the beginning of a new chapter, that will be challenging but also filled with opportunities to connect, to grow, and find meaning in moments you may not expect. Knowledge is power, and understanding what Dementia is—and what it is not—is the first step toward reclaiming a sense of control in a situation that can feel anything but.

As we move forward in this book, we'll explore how to navigate this journey with resilience and love, armed with the knowledge that, even when life turns upside down, there is still beauty in the precious moments that remain.

WHEN TOMORROW FADES:

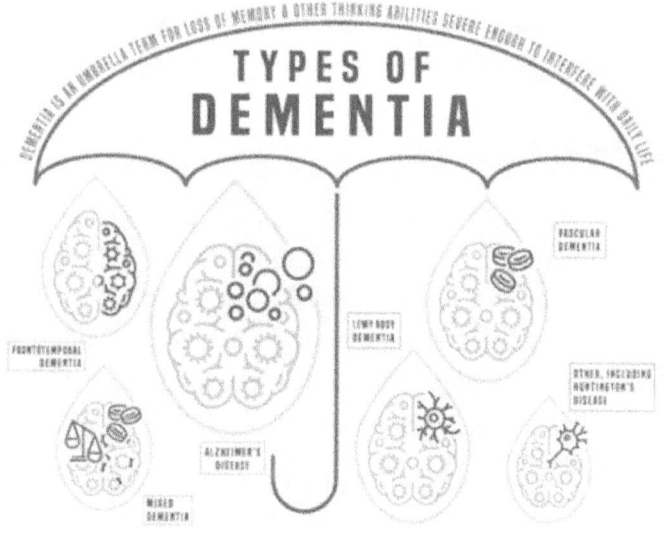

3

How Dementia Changes Your Loved One and Yourself - Unraveling the Puzzle

Caring for a loved one with Dementia is often described as trying to solve a puzzle with missing pieces. Just when you think you've figured out how the pieces fit, the picture shifts, and new gaps appear. This journey is one of constant adjustment, requiring patience, compassion, and a willingness to see beyond the surface of the disease. To begin understanding how Dementia changes your loved one, it helps to step into their world for a moment.

Imagine a Day in the Life of someone with Dementia

This is often the daily reality for someone living with Dementia. While every individual's experience is unique, there are certain symptoms and behaviors which commonly occur at different stages of the disease:

Early Stage: In the beginning, the changes might be subtle. Your loved one might misplace items, struggle to find the right words, or forget appointments. They may feel frustrated or embarrassed by these lapses, leading to anger outbursts or silence. You may also find the milk in the pantry and the car keys in the freezer—a treasure hunt you never signed up for.

Middle Stage: As the disease progresses, memory loss deepens, and confusion becomes more pronounced. You might notice your loved one repeating questions, getting lost in familiar places, or struggling with tasks they once mastered. Personality changes can emerge—a once patient person might become quick to anger, or a reserved individual might grow unusually outgoing. Communication becomes more challenging as words and ideas slip away, leading to frustration for everyone. Be prepared for surprises, like them insisting the dog needs a bath when you don't even have a dog.

Late Stage: In the later stages, the disease affects nearly every aspect of daily life. Your loved one might lose the ability to recognize even close family members. They may require help with basic tasks like eating, dressing, and using the bathroom. At this stage, nonverbal communication often becomes more important—a smile, a gentle touch, or a soothing tone of voice can convey more than words ever could. And don't be surprised if you become their new favorite stranger—a role you didn't audition for but will play with grace.

How your loved one behaves' is your Window into the Disease

One of the most challenging aspects of Dementia is understanding the behaviors that come with it. A loved one who once prided themselves on neatness might start hoarding seemingly random objects. Someone who was always easygoing might become suspicious or accusatory. These changes can be bewildering, even hurtful, but it's crucial to remember one thing: these behaviors are symptoms of the disease, not a reflection of intent or made to hurt you.

Dementia damages the brain's ability to process information and regulate emotions. When your loved one lashes out, refuses to cooperate, or behaves in irrational ways, they are not acting out of malice. They are responding to a world that no longer makes sense to them. Their actions are often driven by fear, frustration, or unmet needs they can no longer articulate. So when they accuse you of stealing their favorite slippers (while they're wearing them), inhale take a deep breath, and remind yourself it's the disease talking.

Recognizing Needs Beyond Symptoms

While Dementia changes many things, it does not erase your loved one's soul. Beneath the confusion and memory loss, they still have feelings, likes and dislikes, and a need for connection. Your role as a caregiver is to manage their symptoms and keep them safe, while recognizing and meeting their deeper needs.

Here are some ways to do that:

Stay Present: Even if they don't remember your name, they feel your presence. A warm smile, a kind word, or simply holding their hand can provide all the comfort and reassurance they need.

Create a Routine: Familiarity provides a sense of security. Simple routines—meals delivered, a favorite song in the morning, or a walk in the garden—can help ground them in a world that to them, often feels chaotic. (And if the same song on repeat drives you a little batty, remember—it's cheaper than therapy.)

Change how you talk: As their language skills decline, look for other ways to connect. Pay attention to body language, tone of voice, and facial expressions. Music, art, or even a favorite scent can evoke memories and emotions when words fail. Sometimes, singing off-key to an old favorite tune can do wonders for both of you.

Focus on Their Strengths: While Dementia takes away certain abilities, it often leaves others intact. Your loved one might still enjoy folding laundry, arranging flowers, or listening to a favorite story. These small tasks can give them a sense of purpose and joy—and folding towels together might become your new meditative practice.

Your Reactions: Finding Grace in the Challenges

It's natural to feel overwhelmed, frustrated, or even resentful. Caring for someone with Dementia is a deeply emotional journey, and your reactions are part of the process. But as you navigate this path, try to extend the same love to yourself that you offer to your loved one.

When their behavior feels particularly challenging, pause and ask yourself: What might they be trying to communicate? Are they hungry, tired, or in pain? Are they scared or overstimulated? Understanding the root of their actions can help you respond with empathy rather than frustration. And if all else fails, remember the golden rule of care giving: laugh when you can and cry when you need to—sometimes both at the same time.

Above all, remember that you are not alone. Support is available—from friends, family, caregivers, and professionals who understand the complexities of this journey. Together, you can unravel the puzzle, one piece at a time, and find moments of connection and love that shine through the haze of Dementia.

First Steps now you have a Diagnosis

A Dementia diagnosis can feel like stepping into a storm without an umbrella. But before the panic sets in, take a deep breath. The key to navigating this journey is preparation, and the first steps involve building a solid foundation of support, organizing essential affairs, and creating a plan to guide you through the ups and downs.

Building a Support Network and Getting Help

Caring for a loved one with Dementia is not a solo mission. One of your first priorities should be assembling a team of allies—family, friends, medical professionals, and support groups. Here are some ways to start:

- *Family and Friends*: Reach out to those closest to you. Even if they can't provide hands-on care, they might be able to offer emotional support or help with errands and appointments.
- *Support Groups*: Joining a Dementia caregiver support group can provide invaluable advice, camaraderie, and understanding from others who've been in your shoes.
- *Professional Help*: Consider hiring a care manager or consulting with a social worker who specializes in elder care to help you navigate the maze of resources and services.

Organizing Legal and Financial Affairs

Taking care of legal and financial matters early can save a lot of stress down the road. These steps are vital to ensure that your loved one's wishes are respected and that you're prepared for the financial realities of care giving. Meet with a counselor or legal advisor who will guide you.

What is Capacity? How Does it Matter?

Capacity is a legal term that refers to a person's ability to understand and make decisions. Early in the disease, while your loved one still has the capacity, it's crucial to address legal and financial planning. Once capacity diminishes, making these decisions becomes much more complicated.

Key Documents to Address:

Power of Attorney (POA): This legal document designates someone to make financial and legal decisions on behalf of your loved one. Without it, even simple tasks like accessing a bank account can become a legal hurdle.

Advance Directives: These documents outline your loved one's preferences for medical care, including end-of-life decisions.

Healthcare Authorizations: HIPAA authorizations ensure that designated individuals -people you select, can access medical information.

What is Guardianship?

Guardianship is a legal arrangement where a court appoints someone to make decisions for an individual who is no longer able to do so and has no one willing to take on this role. While guardianship might be necessary in advanced stages, it's often better to establish a POA early to avoid this more restrictive process.

Understanding Costs of Care and Available Benefits

Caring for someone with Dementia can be expensive, but there are resources to help. Research the costs of care; including in-home services, adult day programs, and long-term care facilities. Look into benefits like Medicaid, veterans' benefits, and long-term care insurance. A financial planner specializing in elder care can be an invaluable resource. Some caregivers must continue to work so what will this look like, who can help?

Planning for Future Transitions

It's important to consider your loved one's evolving needs. Will they stay at home with assistance, or is a memory care facility a better option? Explore these choices early, visit facilities, and discuss preferences with your loved one while they can still share their thoughts.

Creating a Care Plan

Having a care plan is like having a road map for an unpredictable journey. While it won't eliminate surprises, it will provide structure and direction.

Establishing a Daily Routine

Routine is comforting for individuals with Dementia. Consistent meal times, activities, and rest periods can reduce confusion and anxiety. Incorporate meaningful activities like listening to music, gardening, or browsing old photo albums.

Tracking Medical Needs and Medications

Maintain a detailed record of doctor appointments, medications, and any changes in symptoms. A simple notebook or a care giving app can help you stay organized.

Preparing for the Progression of the Disease

Dementia is a slow-moving condition with periods of stability and sudden changes. Learn to e
  educate yourself about what to expect and be prepared to adapt

as needs evolve. Flexibility is key, as are moments of humor to lighten the load. When the toaster ends up in the fridge, remember—it's okay to laugh.

Where to Learn More

Knowledge is power. Equip yourself with information to feel more confident and prepared. Some valuable resources include:

Alzheimer's Association: Offers a wealth of information on all types of Dementia, including local resources and support groups.

Books and Online Courses: Many care giving guides and workshops are available to help you learn practical skills.

Healthcare Providers: Your loved one's doctor or neurologist can recommend reputable resources and specialists.

Community Organizations: Local senior centers, libraries, and nonprofits often host educational events and support programs.

Taking these first steps may feel overwhelming, but remember: every journey begins with a single step. You're building the foundation for a care plan that will guide you and your loved one through this challenging, and meaningful chapter of life.

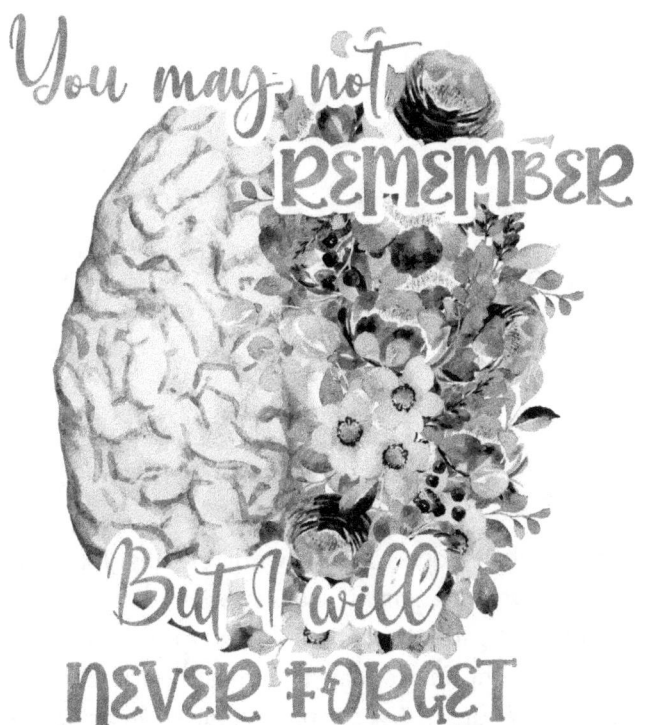

4

Navigating the Maze of What Comes Next?

Caring for a loved one with Dementia can feel like walking through an ever-changing maze. Just when you think you've found the right path, the walls shift, and a new route appears. The key is learning how to adapt and adjust with grace, patience, and a sense of humor. Let's explore some strategies for what comes next.

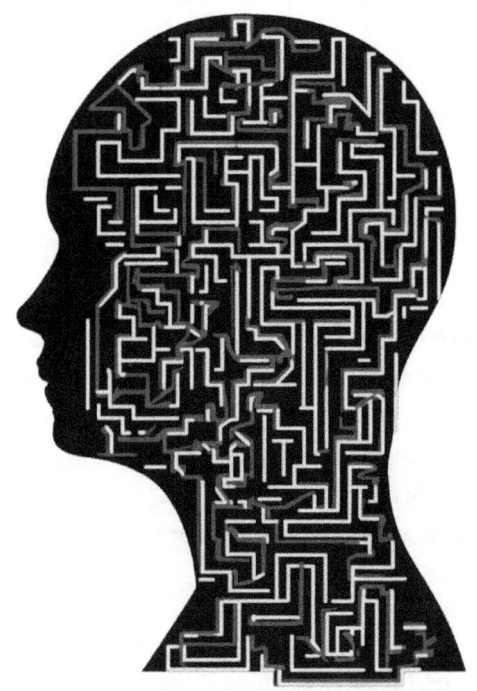

Changing How You Communicate

Communication is a cornerstone of connection, but Dementia changes how your loved one understands and expresses themselves. Adjusting your approach can make a world of difference.

How to Have a Great Conversation with Your Loved One

Start by meeting them where they are. Focus on the present moment, and keep your tone warm and inviting. Here's how:

- Use Short, Simple Sentences: using long and complicated sentences can overwhelm them. Break your thoughts into smaller pieces and speak slowly. Try not to talk as though they are a child but DO use words that are easy to understand, simple and direct.
- Nonverbal Cues: Smiles, gentle touches, and eye contact can communicate more than words.
- Patience is Key: When confusion or frustration arises, take a deep breath and slow down.
- What to Say and What Not to Say
- Do Say: Simple affirmations like, "It's okay," "I'm here," or "Let's do this together."
- Don't Say: "Don't you remember?" or "We just talked about this." These phrases can heighten anxiety and confusion and can make them angry.

Responding Calmly to Agitation or Repetitive Behaviors

When your loved one repeats a question for the tenth time, remember: that they're not doing it on purpose. Respond with calm reassurance. Redirection can also help—guide them toward an activity or topic that soothes them.

Understanding Triggers and Behaviors

Dementia behaviors are a form of communication, often as a result of unmet needs or environmental triggers.

Identifying and Minimizing Triggers

Common Triggers: Loud noises, unfamiliar settings, or changes in routine.

Solutions: Create a calm, predictable environment. Stick to routines and minimize distractions.

Redirecting Attention

When confusion or aggression arises, try shifting focus to something calming, like music, a favorite hobby, or looking through old photos. Distraction can be a powerful tool.

Accepting Behaviors as Communication

Rather than viewing behaviors as problems, see them as your loved one's way of expressing a need. Are they hungry, thirsty, tired, or in pain? Looking beyond the behavior can help you respond with empathy. **The anger they show sometimes is hard to take when you know you're doing everything possible to care for them.**

Maintaining Connection

Even as Dementia progresses, moments of connection are still possible and deeply meaningful. Keep a journal or diary to remind you of the good moments. An affirmation diary can also be helpful for those days when you just can't find the light.

Finding Joy in Small Shared Moments

A shared laugh, holding hands, or enjoying a sunny day together can bring joy. Celebrate these moments.

Using Music, Photos, and Stories

Familiar tunes, cherished photographs, and storytelling can spark recognition and comfort. Music, in particular, has a remarkable way of reaching those with Dementia. Recordings of songs are never easier to locate with online apps and music download.

Adjusting Expectations While Preserving Dignity

Your loved one may no longer remember your name, but they can feel your love. Shift your focus to their current abilities while respecting their need for autonomy and dignity.

Managing Daily Care and Making Your Home Safe

Practical adjustments to your environment and care giving routines can make life easier for everyone.

- Reduce Fall Risks: Remove loose rugs, install grab bars, and ensure good lighting.
- "Loved One" Proofing: Secure sharp objects, cleaning supplies, and medications.
- Easy Eating and Drinking Tips: Use non-slip plates and cups, and offer finger foods if utensils are challenging.
- You may need door locks to keep them safe if they wander
- Mobility ramps can be portable, temporary, or permanent

Creating Dementia-Friendly Spaces

- Labels and Signage: Clearly label drawers, doors, and everyday items to reduce confusion.
- Simplify the Environment: Keep decor minimal and free of clutter.
- Lighting Matters: Ensure rooms are well-lit to reduce shadows and confusion.

Maintaining Familiar Surroundings

Familiarity brings comfort. Keeping the environment consistent and predictable can reduce anxiety and promote a sense of security.

Assisting with Personal Care

Personal care tasks can be challenging but are opportunities to maintain your loved one's dignity and comfort.

- Techniques for Bathing and Dressing can be found online through YouTube or by contacting your local Senior Center or Home Health.
- Bathing: It should be relaxing, with warm water, soft towels, and calm reassurance.
- Dressing: Lay-out clothing in the order it should be put on, and offer simple choices to maintain independence.

Encouraging Eating and Hydration

- Serve small, manageable portions. A normal-sized plate from the past will be too much - they will then eat nothing being overwhelmed.
- Offer favorite foods, with lots of color, and keep water accessible throughout the day.
- Don't change how you cook. Remember you too must eat. Prepare your meals and then blend their meal making it softer. Cooking should not become a chore.

Monitoring and Managing Incontinence

Incontinence is common but manageable. Use protective bedding, pads can be bought cheaply at the pet store (much cheaper than medical issues) they are the same!! Take them to the bathroom on a schedule, and use a matter-of-fact attitude to reduce embarrassment for you both.

Balancing Independence and Assistance

Striking the right balance between helping and encouraging independence is essential. Don't rush to help because they are too slow let them take their time.

Encouraging Participation

Involve your loved one in tasks they can still manage, like folding laundry or stirring ingredients. These activities provide a sense of purpose. People with Dementia thrive with repetition. They will fold laundry for hours so let them fold, then mess them up for the person to begin again. This will be much harder on you than them. I have seen people spend hours on laundry.

Knowing When to Step In

Be observant. Step in gently when frustration builds or safety is at risk.

Adapting Tasks to Their Abilities

Break down activities into smaller steps and simplify where needed. Focus on what they can do rather than what they've lost.

Navigating the maze of Dementia care giving is challenging, with adaptability, creativity, and a strong foundation of love and support, it's possible to create a journey filled with connection and meaning.

5

Recognizing the Signs of Late-Stage Dementia

As the disease and time progresses, changes become more pronounced, and your role as a caregiver will shift significantly. This can be one of the hardest parts of the journey, but understanding what to expect can help you prepare emotionally, physically, and practically.

Physical and Cognitive Changes

As Dementia progresses, the body and mind undergo profound changes:

Loss of Mobility and Increased Frailty: Your loved one may spend more time in bed or a chair, as moving around becomes difficult. Muscles weaken, and the balance becomes unsteady despite all the food, and exercise you may have been offering.

Severe Memory Loss and Minimal Communication: Recognizing even close family members might fade, and verbal communication may be reduced to just a few words or sounds. Eye contact or facial expressions become the primary way they connect - focus on their face.

Increased Dependence on Caregivers: At this stage, your loved one will rely on you for all their needs—feeding, dressing, bathing, and more. This can feel overwhelming, but take it one moment at a time.

Health Complications to Expect

Late-stage Dementia brings certain health challenges you'll need to watch for:

Risk of Infections:

Your loved one becomes more prone to infections like pneumonia or urinary tract infections (Ut Is). Watch for fevers, changes in behavior, or signs of pain. These can happen despite all the precautions you may be taking again you have not failed them!

Difficulty Swallowing and Eating:

Eating and drinking may become harder as swallowing reflexes weaken. Soft foods, thickened liquids, and small, manageable bites can help. Protein shakes, soup, put food into the blender to soften. Cook your regular meals do not change your diet, then simply blend the meal for them. This will save on waste, and help you maintain your health and eat the foods you love.

Changes in Sleep Patterns and Energy Levels:

Your loved one may sleep much more during the day and seem less responsive. This is part of the body slowing down. They may also be up all night. We call this sundowning. Leave lights on in the house to help with this as their personal time clock has become altered.

Emotional and Spiritual Preparation

The emotional toll of this stage can be immense, but there are ways to find comfort and meaning:

Coping with Anticipatory Grief:

Grieving begins long before the final goodbye. Allow yourself to feel the sadness, frustration, and love. Lean on friends, family, or a counselor for support. Connect with your church or even a local Bereavement counselor they can be very helpful at this stage as you are grieving the loss of the person you knew even before they pass away.

Creating a Space for Meaningful Goodbyes:

This can be a time to share stories, play favorite music, or sit in silence. Even if your loved one can't respond, they will feel your love. Big box stores and Amazon have plaster kits you can buy to make hand prints for remembrance. Making their favorite clothes into dolls or a comfort cushion. There are many great ideas on Etsy or Pinterest.

Honoring Their Emotional and Spiritual Needs:

Through faith, music, rituals, or personal reflection, find ways to bring peace and comfort in their final days.

Transitioning to End-of-Life Care

End-of-life decisions are never easy, but they are a natural part of this journey. Your love and care will help guide you through this time.

Now You Have Made the Decision to Keep Them at Home....

Assessing Your Capacity to Provide Care: Can you manage the physical, emotional, and practical demands of end-of-life care? It's okay to admit if you need help. Home Health can help for a short period to help you learn to manage your loved one safely, things like bathing, lifting, and transferring from bed to chair have skills you will need to keep yourself safe and prevent injury.

Balancing Medical Needs with Their Wishes: Talk with doctors and family members about your loved one's care preferences. Would they feel most at peace at home, or is professional care a better fit?

Knowing When Professional Help Is Needed: It's not a failure to ask for help. Whether it's hiring home care or transitioning to a care facility, the goal is always your loved one's comfort and dignity.

Engaging Hospice and Palliative Care Services

Hospice care can be a lifeline for both your loved one and you during this stage:

- What Hospice Care Provides: Hospice focuses on comfort rather than cure, offering pain management, emotional support, and help for the entire family. Know they do not take over from the family. If you are struggling with no support they can help guide you in determining where the best place is for your loved one to live if you can't maintain them at home. Their social workers have great resources.
- Managing Pain and Discomfort: Hospice professionals are trained to ensure your loved one remains as pain-free and comfortable as possible.
- Communicating with Doctors and Hospice Staff: Ask questions, express concerns, and share your loved one's wishes. Clear communication ensures the best care.

Providing Emotional Comfort

In these final days, your presence matters more than ever. Even when words fail, love remains.

- Using Touch, Music, and Presence: A gentle hand on theirs, a soft song, or simply sitting close can offer deep reassurance.
- Creating a Peaceful, Soothing Environment: Keep the room quiet and calm—soft lighting, familiar objects, and gentle music can create a comforting space.
- Preserving Dignity and Love: Treat your loved one with the same care and respect you always have. Small gestures, like brushing their hair or speaking to them kindly, show that they are still valued and love

While late-stage Dementia is a time of profound change, it is also a time for love, reflection, and presence. You may feel like you are navigating uncharted waters, but remember—you are not alone. **Lean** on support systems, care professionals, and your inner strength as you walk this final part of the journey together.

WHEN TOMORROW FADES:

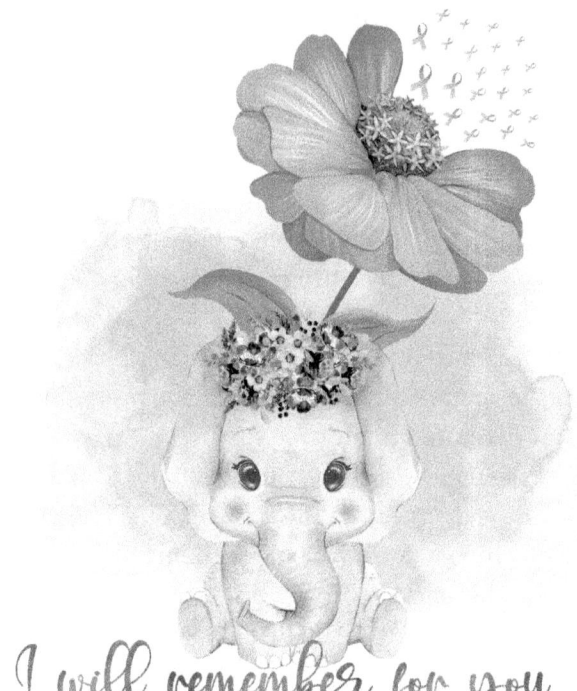

6

Honoring Caregivers'

There are over 45 million caregivers in the world, and 11 million* in the United States alone providing unpaid care to a loved one living with Dementia every day. That is a staggering number. Every year approximately 10 million families are given this dreaded news and diagnosis. Being trusted to deliver care is a role born of love and loyalty, and while often a necessity it's a labor of the heart—but let's be honest, it's also exhausting. Between managing appointments, tracking medications, and trying to keep your loved one calm, it's easy to forget about someone else who desperately needs your attention: **YOU!**

You can't pour from an empty cup, and if you're not careful, care giving can leave you feeling depleted, resentful, or struggling with health issues. This chapter is about you—how to care for yourself while caring for your loved one and how to find that elusive balance between their needs and your own life.

Why Self-Care Matters

Imagine your loved one relies on you as their safety-net—solid, steady, and dependable. But what happens if you start to fray? The truth is, you're only human. Care giving without taking care of yourself is like driving a car on empty: eventually, you'll break down.

Taking care of yourself doesn't mean you're selfish, lazy, or ignoring your loved one. It's the opposite—it's what allows you to show up for them, day after day, with love and energy. Self-care isn't a luxury; it's a necessity. When you care for yourself, you care for them better.

Recognizing Stress (And What It Does to You)

Care giving stress doesn't always mirror the dramatic moments we see in movies. It can be sneaky. It's the irritability when your loved one asks the same question for the 15th time. It's the guilt you feel when you lose your patience. It's lying awake at night, worrying about tomorrow.

Chronic stress can lead to physical and emotional issues like:

- Exhaustion and trouble sleeping
- Anxiety, depression, and feeling overwhelmed
- Frequent headaches, stomach issues, or body aches
- Forgetfulness, trouble concentrating, and burnout

Recognizing these signs is the first step to overcoming them. You're not failing as a caregiver; you're just running on fumes. **It's time to refuel.**

Practical Self-Care Strategies

Self-care doesn't have to be a weekend getaway to a spa (though that does sound nice). It can be small, intentional actions you incorporate into your day to protect your well-being:

- Take Small Breaks: A 10-minute walk outside, five minutes of deep breathing, or a cup of coffee in peace can reset your mind.
- Ask for Help: Repeat after me: I cannot do this alone. And you shouldn't have to. Call on friends, family, or professional respite care services to give you regular breaks.
- Say "Yes" to What Nourishes You: Whether reading, gardening, painting, or dancing to your favorite music—find an activity that feels like you and schedule it regularly.
- Say "No" Without Guilt: You can't take on everything. It's okay to set boundaries with others (and yourself) and prioritize what matters.
- Stay Connected: Care giving can feel isolating, so make time to connect with friends, a support group, or someone who "gets it." Even a quick phone call can lighten the load.
- Move Your Body: Exercise doesn't have to be intense. A walk, gentle stretching, or yoga can help relieve stress and improve your energy.
- Take Care of Your Health: Don't skip doctor's appointments, eat regularly, and get as much rest as possible. Your health

is just as important as your loved one's.

Balancing Caregiving and Your Personal Life

Balancing your caregiving role with your personal life isn't easy—it's a juggling act. Some days, you'll drop a ball or two. That's okay. But creating a balance starts with setting priorities and realistic expectations:

- Define What Balance Means to You: Balance doesn't mean equal attention all the time to everything. It means finding time for the things that matter—your family, your hobbies, your career—while meeting your loved one's needs.
- Schedule "Me Time": Put it on your calendar like an appointment. Even 20 minutes of personal time can make a difference.
- Set Boundaries: Learn to say "no" when you need to. You don't have to take every phone call, respond to every message, or attend every event.
- Lean on Others: Let others share the load. Whether it's help from family, friends, or professional caregivers, don't be afraid to delegate tasks so you can breathe.
- Remember Who You Are Outside of Caregiving: You're still you—a partner, a parent, a friend, an artist, a dreamer. Don't let caregiving define your entire identity.

HONORING CAREGIVERS'

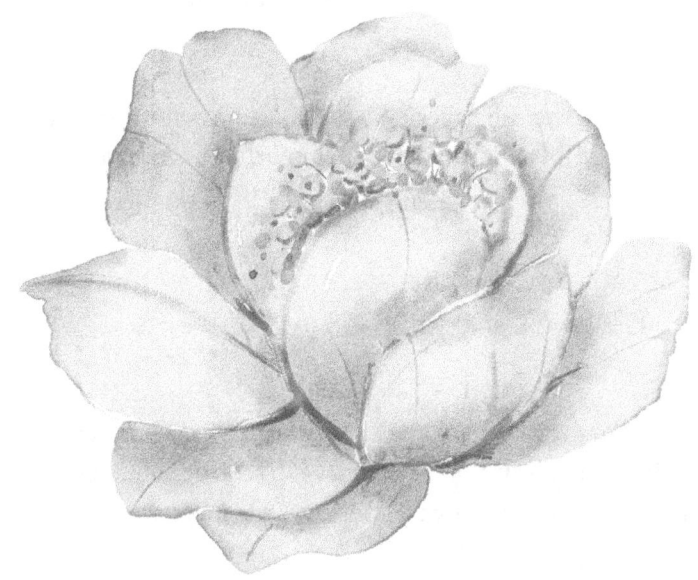

When You Feel Overwhelmed

There will be moments when it feels too much—when the tears won't stop or your patience wears thin. That's normal. On days like this, pause and remind yourself:

- You are doing the best you can.
- It's okay to ask for help.
- It's okay to feel tired, angry, sad, or frustrated.

When overwhelm strikes, step back. Take a deep breath, cry if you need to, and lean on your support network. You are not alone.

You Deserve Care, Too

Caring for a loved one is one of the most selfless things you can do. But that doesn't mean you have to sacrifice yourself in the process. You are worthy of care, love, and joy, too.

So, as you navigate this challenging yet meaningful journey, remember to care for you. Because when you're healthy, rested, and supported, you can show up for your loved one with a full heart—and that makes all the difference.

With love and a gentle reminder to be kind to yourself, from
    The Author Who Believes in You

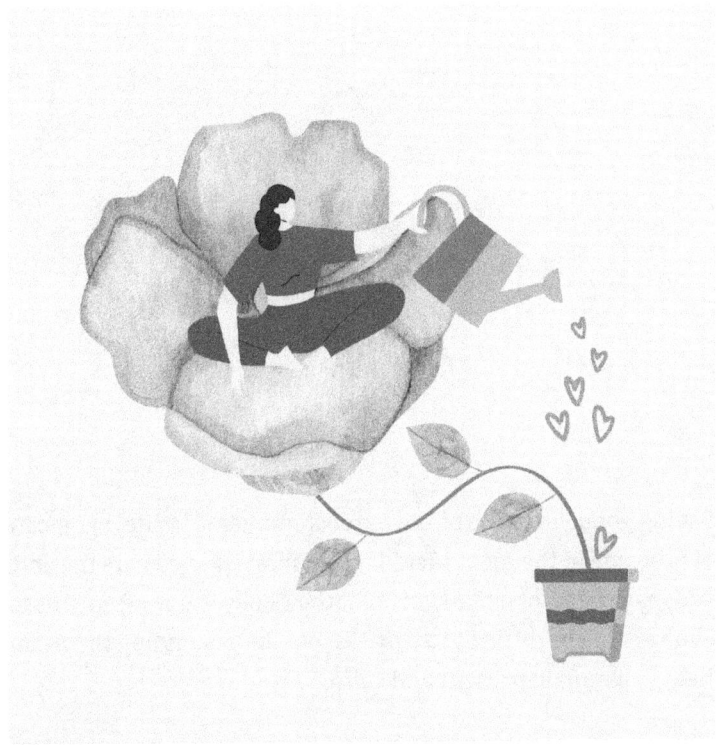

The journey with Dementia doesn't end with your loved one's passing. What comes next is just as important—the space where love, grief, and healing intertwine. This final chapter is about honoring the life that was, finding peace, and rediscovering yourself in a world forever changed.

7

The Final Goodbye

Saying goodbye is one of the hardest moments in life, yet it can also be one of the most sacred. As your loved one nears the end, you may begin to notice signs that their body is letting go. These changes can be difficult to witness, but understanding them can help you remain present and calm.

Recognizing End-of-Life Symptoms

- Changes in Breathing, Circulation, and Alertness: You may notice irregular breathing, long pauses, or a softening of their energy. Hands and feet may feel cooler as circulation slows. They may become less responsive, retreating inward.

- What to Expect During the Final Moments: The body will

gradually shut down. Breaths may slow, and there may be a sense of peaceful stillness. It's not uncommon to feel their spirit begin to slip away before the body fully does. Know that this process is natural—and you are there to ease their passage with love.

- Staying Present and Calm: Your presence matters more than you realize. Hold their hand, play soft music, or whisper words of comfort. Let them know they are loved, and it's okay to let go. Your calm can be a gift in their final moments.

Honoring Their Legacy

After the goodbye comes the remembering. Your loved one's story is far greater than their illness, and honoring that truth can bring comfort.

- Memorializing Your Loved One: Whether it's through a celebration of life, a quiet ceremony, or planting a tree in their honor, find a way to say goodbye that feels right to you.

- Celebrating Their Life Beyond Their Illness: Dementia may

have been part of their journey, but it doesn't define who they were. Share stories of their humor, kindness, quirks, and passions. Keep the focus on their life—not just their loss.

- Involving Family and Friends: Grief can feel isolating, but you are not alone. Encourage family and friends to share memories, laughter, and tears. Connection can be the balm that begins to heal the wounds.

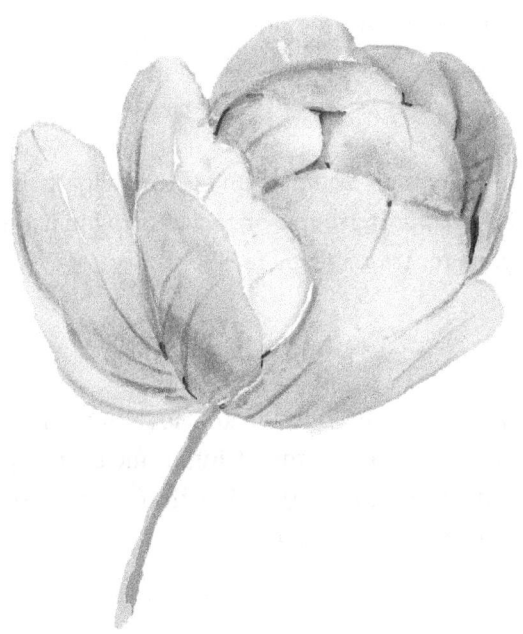

Grieving and Healing

Grief is not a straight path; it ebbs and flows like a tide. It will change over time, but it never fully disappears—because love never does.

- Understanding Grief Is Non-Linear: You may find yourself fine one moment and sobbing the next. That's okay. Grief has no timeline and no rules.

- Finding Support: You don't have to navigate grief alone. Therapy, support groups, or even writing in a journal can help you process what you feel.

- Giving Yourself Permission to Move Forward: Moving forward doesn't mean forgetting. It means carrying your loved one with you as you step into the future. You can honor their life by living yours fully.

Rebuilding Your Life After Care giving

For so long, your days have been shaped by the needs of someone else. Now, you face a new question: *Who am I now?* Rebuilding your life after care giving can feel like learning to walk again—but it's also a chance to rediscover yourself.

Rediscovering Your Own Identity

Adjusting to Life Without the Caregiver Role: It's okay to feel lost at first. Your role as a caregiver has ended, but you are still *you*. Take time to breathe, to rest, and to feel your way forward.

Exploring New Hobbies, Goals, or Relationships: Maybe there's a book you've always wanted to write, a class you've wanted to take, or a place you've wanted to visit. Now is the time to explore the things that bring you joy.

Allowing Time and Space for Reflection: This new chapter is not a race. Give yourself the grace to look inward, to reflect on where you've been, and to dream about where you want to go.

Maintaining Your Connection with Them

Your loved one may be gone, but the bond you share doesn't have to end.

Keeping Their Memory Alive: Talk about them often. Hang their favorite photo, play their favorite music, or cook a meal they loved. These small rituals can keep their spirit close.

Sharing Their Stories with Future Generations: Tell their grandchildren about their jokes, their kindness, or their love of dancing in the kitchen. Stories are the thread that keeps them part of your family's fabric.

Finding Peace in Their Legacy: Whether it's through quiet reflection or honoring their wishes, find comfort in knowing their life touched yours and made it richer.

Helping Others on the Journey

One of the most meaningful ways to heal is to help others walking the same path.

Supporting Other Caregivers: Share what you've learned—the tips, the hard days, and the love that got you through. Your experience can be a lifeline for someone else.

Volunteering or Advocating for Dementia Causes: Whether it's raising awareness, participating in a fundraiser, or volunteering at a memory care center, your involvement can make a difference.

Turning Your Journey Into Strength: This experience has changed you. It has made you stronger, wiser, and more compassionate. Take that strength and use it to light the way for others.

8

Conclusion: A Journey of Love, Laughter, and Purpose

Congratulations you have made it. As we reach the final pages of this book, I want you to take a deep breath, pour yourself a cup of tea, and give yourself a pat on the back. You've shown up whether you're just beginning this journey, knee-deep in it, or looking back with a heart full of love and memories. More than any perfect plan, strategy, or system, being there and being you is what your loved one needs most.

Your Loved One Needs You

Dementia is an uninvited guest who barges in, shuffling the furniture, stealing memories, and turning everything upside down. But while the disease changes so much, it cannot steal the bond you share with your loved one. You are their anchor in a stormy sea, their familiar face when the world feels unrecognizable. Your presence—your patience, your touch, your smile—is what brings comfort when words fail. And when you feel like you've run out of everything—energy, tears, patience—remember: the love you're giving matters more than you'll ever know.

Of course, you're human. You'll mess up. You'll snap when you shouldn't. You'll cry when you thought you'd hold it together. That's okay. Forgive yourself, laugh where you can, and keep showing up. Because love is not about being perfect—it's about being present.

Finding Your Purpose in This New Reality

As life changes and care giving becomes part of your identity, it's easy to feel lost. Who are you now? What happened to the person you were before? The truth is, care giving changes you—but it doesn't erase you. It gives you a new purpose, shaped by resilience, compassion, and a strength you probably didn't know you had. This journey may not be the one you signed up for, but it can bring depth, meaning, and yes, even joy!

Your purpose will shift as you go. Maybe today it's as simple as making your loved one smile today. Tomorrow might mean finding a support group, asking for help, or caring for yourself for a change. And one day, when you look back on this chapter, you'll realize you grew, too. You've become stronger, wiser, and deeply loving through the tough days and tender moments, you've become stronger, wiser, and deeply loving.

Carrying Their Light Forward

This book has walked you through the ups and downs of Dementia care giving—the confusion, the heartbreak, the laughter, and the unexpected beauty of it all. And as you continue forward, know that your story doesn't end here. Even after that final goodbye, your loved one's light stays with you. You carry their smile in your own, their laugh in your heart, and their spirit in how you show up for others.

So, my dear reader, thank you for walking this path with me. If this book brought you comfort, hope, or maybe even a little chuckle during a hard moment, I'd be honored if you shared your thoughts in a review on Amazon. Your words might help another caregiver feel seen, understood, and a little less alone.

Final Thoughts

Dementia may have taken so much, but it cannot take away the love you shared, the memories you cherish, or the person you have become through this journey. Your role as a caregiver was a testament to your strength and love—a beautiful, selfless act that will forever remain a part of you.

As you step into what comes next, know this: You carry your loved one with you. They live on in your laughter, in your stories, and in the quiet moments when you feel their presence. This is not the end; it's simply a continuation—a legacy of love that never fades.

A Caregiver's Heart

In quiet moments, you stand so strong,
When days feel endless, and nights are long.
A gentle touch, a patient word,
Your love is steady, seen and heard.

Though memories fade, and time moves on,
You are the light when the way feels gone.
With every smile, with every care,
You give them comfort, you're always there.

So take a breath, and know it's true—
The work you do has meaning too.
A heart like yours, so brave, so kind,
is the greatest gift a soul can find.

I understand what you are going through, the struggle, the emotional turmoil, the pain, and countless sacrifices. I hope this book is helpful to you as you journey with your loved one.

If you liked this book please leave a review on Amazon.
Please remember, to always be kind to yourself.
Pam D Moore

9

Resources

Alzheimer Disease International https://www.alzint.org/

https://www.etsy.com/

memorybridge. (2009, May 26). Gladys Wilson and Naomi Feil [Video]. YouTube. https://www.youtube.com/watch?v=CrZXz10FcVM

https://www.pinterest.com/deborahdrapac/alzheimers-activities/

UCLA Dementia Caregiver Training: Agitation and Anxiety | UCLA Alzheimer's and Dementia Care Program https://www.youtube.com/watch?v=hahvUXwTXE4

World Alzheimer's Day is celebrated on September 21st each year.

www.ingramcontent.com/pod-product-compliance
Lightning Source LLC
Chambersburg PA
CBHW070414230526
45471CB00006B/2795